Cambridge Elements ☰

Elements in Emergency Neurosurgery
edited by
Nihal Gurusinghe
Lancashire Teaching Hospital NHS Trust
Peter Hutchinson
University of Cambridge, Society of British Neurological Surgeons and Royal College of Surgeons of England
Ioannis Fouyas
Royal College of Surgeons of Edinburgh
Naomi Slator
North Bristol NHS Trust
Ian Kamaly-Asl
Royal Manchester Children's Hospital
Peter Whitfield
University Hospitals Plymouth NHS Trust

CRANIAL AND SPINAL TUBERCULOSIS INFECTIONS INCLUDING ACUTE PRESENTATIONS

Veekshith Shetty
Manipal Hospital, Bangalore

Pragnesh Bhatt
Aberdeen Royal Infirmary

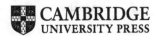

CAMBRIDGE
UNIVERSITY PRESS

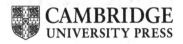

Shaftesbury Road, Cambridge CB2 8EA, United Kingdom

One Liberty Plaza, 20th Floor, New York, NY 10006, USA

477 Williamstown Road, Port Melbourne, VIC 3207, Australia

314–321, 3rd Floor, Plot 3, Splendor Forum, Jasola District Centre, New Delhi – 110025, India

103 Penang Road, #05–06/07, Visioncrest Commercial, Singapore 238467

Cambridge University Press is part of Cambridge University Press & Assessment, a department of the University of Cambridge.

We share the University's mission to contribute to society through the pursuit of education, learning and research at the highest international levels of excellence.

www.cambridge.org
Information on this title: www.cambridge.org/9781009517324

DOI: 10.1017/9781009388764

When citing this work, please include a reference to the DOI 10.1017/9781009388764

First published 2024

A catalogue record for this publication is available from the British Library.

ISBN 978-1-009-51732-4 Hardback
ISBN 978-1-009-38873-3 Paperback
ISSN 2755-0656 (online)
ISSN 2755-0648 (print)

Cambridge University Press & Assessment has no responsibility for the persistence or accuracy of URLs for external or third-party internet websites referred to in this publication and does not guarantee that any content on such websites is, or will remain, accurate or appropriate.

Every effort has been made in preparing this Element to provide accurate and up-to-date information which is in accord with accepted standards and practice at the time of publication. Although case histories are drawn from actual cases, every effort has been made to disguise the identities of the individuals involved. Nevertheless, the authors, editors and publishers can make no warranties that the information contained herein is totally free from error, not least because clinical standards are constantly changing through research and regulation. The authors, editors and publishers therefore disclaim all liability for direct or consequential damages resulting from the use of material contained in this Element. Readers are strongly advised to pay careful attention to information provided by the manufacturer of any drugs or equipment that they plan to use.

Cranial and Spinal Tuberculosis Infections including Acute Presentations

Elements in Emergency Neurosurgery

DOI: 10.1017/9781009388764
First published online: April 2024

Veekshith Shetty
Manipal Hospital, Bangalore

Pragnesh Bhatt
Aberdeen Royal Infirmary

Author for correspondence: Veekshith Shetty, shetty699@gmail.com

Abstract: Central nervous system affliction, although rare, represents one of the most severe extra-pulmonary manifestations of tuberculosis (TB), potentially leading to substantial morbidity and mortality if not promptly addressed. Cranial TB can manifest in various forms, including tuberculomas, encephalitis, abscesses, and meningitis, with the latter being the most critical and carrying a poor prognosis if left untreated. Spinal TB, accounting for approximately 50% of musculoskeletal TB cases, can present with a spectrum of symptoms, ranging from simple back pain to more severe neurological deficits such as weakness and deformity. Anti-TB medications remain the cornerstone of treatment, and this Element offers an algorithmic approach to managing referrals of suspected TB, incorporating pertinent clinical information to facilitate effective decision-making.

Keywords: spinal tuberculosis, cranial tuberculosis, surgery in spinal tuberculosis, tuberculous meningitis, tuberculomas

ISBNs: 9781009517324 (HB), 9781009388733 (PB), 9781009388764 (OC)
ISSNs: 2755-0656 (online), 2755-0648 (print)

Contents

Introduction

Central nervous system (CNS) tuberculosis (TB) approximately affects 1% of patients with active TB (1). Tuberculosis in the brain most commonly manifests as tuberculous meningitis. Other manifestations of cranial TB include tuberculoma, tuberculous abscess, and encephalopathy. Spinal TB accounts for approximately 50% of musculoskeletal TB burden globally with spinal spondylitis being the most frequent manifestation. Intramedullary tuberculomas and arachnoiditis, although rare, are other notable forms of spinal TB. This Element aims to provide a comprehensive overview of cranial and spinal TB infections, including their pathogenesis, clinical presentation, diagnosis, and management strategies.

1 Cranial Tuberculosis Infection

1.1 Clinical Scenarios

1.1.1 Scenario 1

A 21-year-old male presents to the emergency department with a two-week history of gradually worsening headache accompanied by intermittent low-grade fever. Over the last three days, he has become increasingly drowsy, and his family members have noticed that he has become more confused and disoriented. The patient has no significant past medical history and no known allergies. He is not on any medications. On examination, the patient is drowsy but arousable, confused, and disoriented, and follows simple commands with neck stiffness. There are no focal neurological deficits, and the rest of the systemic examination is normal. Blood samples were sent for routine infectious disease workup, and a magnetic resonance imaging (MRI) of the brain was performed (see Figure 1).

Based on the clinical presentation and radiological findings, what would be the most likely diagnosis?

What additional information would you need to gather to further support this diagnosis? What recommendations would you provide to the referring team?

Under what circumstances would you consider transferring the patient for surgical intervention?

1.1.2 Scenario 2

A 45-year-old female was brought to the emergency department by her husband due to complaints of severe headache, nausea, and vomiting for the past week. The patient also reported a history of intermittent fever, night sweats, and weight loss over the past few months. She originally hails from South Asia and has been living in the United Kingdom for the past 20 years. On examination, she appeared

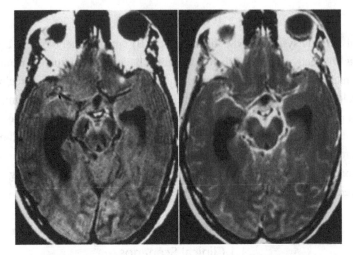

Figure 1 T1 axial and T1 with contrast MRI images

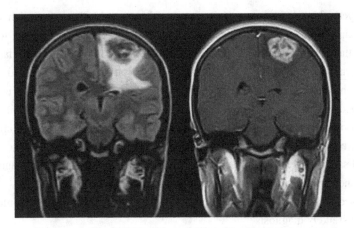

Figure 2 Coronal T2 flair and T1 post contrast images

pale and dehydrated. Her vital signs were within normal limits except for a slightly elevated temperature of 38.2°C. A neurological examination revealed no focal neurological deficits. The rest of the systemic examination was normal. An MRI brain was performed (see Figure 2).

Based on the patient's history and examination, what is the most likely diagnosis?

What investigations would you like to order to confirm the diagnosis?

What is the recommended management for this patient, including medical treatment, follow-up, and potential complications, and what are the key factors to consider in treatment planning and monitoring?

The clinical scenarios presented earlier require a comprehensive understanding of TB to make the most appropriate clinical decision. By reading this Element, an overview of managing such scenarios can be gained, which will enable effective referral and answer the questions posed at the end of each scenario.

1.2 Core Knowledge

1.2.1 Epidemiology

According to the World Health Organization's (WHO) report in 2020, TB ranked as the 13th most prominent cause of mortality and was the second most prevalent infectious disease responsible for fatalities, following COVID-19. Those who contract the TB bacterium face a 5–10% likelihood of developing active TB disease over their lifetime (2). The global prevalence of CNS TB is about 2 per 100,000 inhabitants. The burden of TB in the country, Human Development Index, and the prevalence of human immunodeficiency virus (HIV) are the most important prevalence moderators, especially in patients with TB (3). Tuberculous meningitis is the most common and lethal manifestation of CNS TB.

1.2.2 Pathophysiology

Tuberculosis-related CNS infection primarily occurs through haematogenous dissemination, leading to bacterium deposition within the meninges and subsequent development of caseating necrosis regions, commonly referred to as Rich's foci. This process can promote the subarachnoid dissemination of bacilli (4).

Tuberculous meningitis is characterised by seeding of the bacterium within the cerebrospinal fluid (CSF), resulting in the accumulation of gelatinous exudates primarily within the basal cisterns. This accumulation obstructs the normal CSF circulation and absorption, leading to hydrocephalus. Furthermore, vasculitis of vessels in and around the circle of Willis can promote steno-occlusive changes that may result in stroke or infarction. Chest radiographs reveal that about 50% of patients with tuberculous meningitis have either active or healed pulmonary TB, while 10% have miliary disease, which strongly correlates with CNS involvement (5).

Tuberculomas, often solitary, occur due to continued granuloma growth, consisting of epithelioid and giant cells mixed with predominantly lymphocytes, around a central area of caseating necrosis. Notably, these granulomas usually do not rupture into the subarachnoid space (6).

1.2.3 Clinical Presentation

In cases of tuberculous meningitis, patients typically present with fever accompanied by nocturnal diaphoresis, headache, vomiting, and disorientation. These manifestations may be concomitant with constitutional symptoms, including weight loss, malaise, and anorexia, persisting for a duration of two to four weeks. Several factors can increase an individual's susceptibility to either primary infection or reactivation of latent infection. These factors include immunosuppressed states such as co-infection with HIV (with CD4+ cell counts less than 200 cells/mm^3), chronic alcoholism, stage 4/5 chronic kidney disease, intravenous drug use, poorly controlled diabetes mellitus, malignancy, corticosteroid treatment, and administration of tumour necrosis factor inhibitors. Individuals who have close contact with patients infected with TB, belong to lower socio-economic strata, or have travelled to endemic regions are at an increased risk of acquiring infection.

Cranial neuropathies, predominantly the sixth nerve palsy, and focal neurological deficits are frequently observed on examination. The clinical presentation may be further complicated by the occurrence of seizures (approximately 10–15%, with higher incidence in paediatric patients), hyponatremia (attributable to either cerebral salt wasting (CSW) or syndrome of inappropriate antidiuretic hormone (SIADH) secretion), vasculitis or cerebral infarction (in more than 50%), and hydrocephalus (in approximately 66%), potentially culminating in a comatose state (6).

Clinical manifestations of cerebral tuberculomas, similar to other intracranial mass lesions, primarily depend on the anatomical location of the lesion. Common symptoms include headache, fever, unexplained weight loss, and neurological deficits. Supratentorial lesions may also be associated with seizures in addition to the aforementioned symptoms. Brainstem tuberculomas exhibit long tract signs and multiple cranial nerve dysfunction, whereas cerebellar tuberculomas primarily manifest as gait and balance difficulties. The duration of symptoms typically ranges from weeks to months (7).

Tuberculous abscesses often present more acutely and with rapid deterioration compared to tuberculomas.

1.2.4 Causative Agent

Mycobacterium TB (MTB) is the predominant causative organism, which is an aerobic, non-motile, and non-spore-forming bacterium.

1.3 Clinical Pathway

For a step-by-step guide on diagnosing and managing suspected CNS TB, the following algorithm will be helpful (see Figure 3).

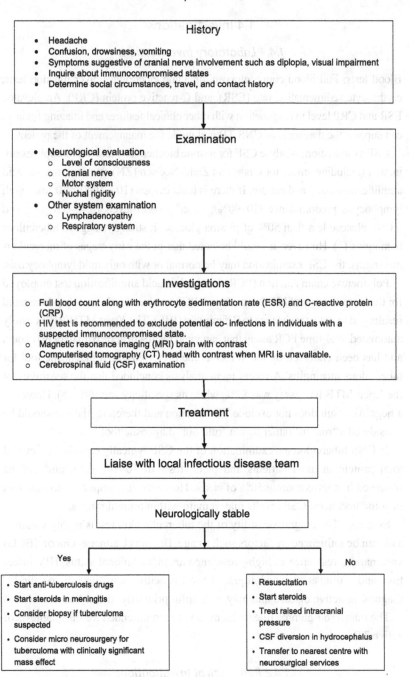

Figure 3 An algorithm for clinical approach to cranial tuberculosis

1.4 Investigations

1.4.1 Laboratory Investigations

Blood tests: Full blood count, glucose, urea and electrolytes, liver function tests, erythrocyte sedimentation rate (ESR), and C-reactive protein (CRP). An elevated ESR and CRP level in conjunction with other clinical features and imaging findings can support the diagnosis of CNS TB and guide the management of the patient.

CSF examination: Analyse CSF for routine biochemistry and microscopic examination (including smear for Gram and Ziehl-Neelsen (ZN) staining), nucleic acid amplification assay and culture. If there is leukocytosis ($10 - 1000 \times 10^3$/mL) with lymphocytic predominance (30–90%), raised protein levels (0.45–3.0 g/L), and a CSF glucose less than 50% of plasma glucose, it strongly suggests tuberculous meningitis (1). However, it should be noted that in the early stages of tuberculous meningitis, the CSF examination may be normal or with only mild lymphocytosis.

Polymerase chain reaction (PCR) is a nucleic acid amplification test employed for the identification of MTB complex. A PCR test has the ability to produce rapid results and to detect resistance to Rifampicin (RIF). The Xpert MTB/RIF is a fully automated, real-time PCR assay that can yield results in approximately two hours and has been endorsed by the WHO as the preferred initial diagnostic tool for tuberculous meningitis. A recent meta-analysis concluded that the sensitivity of the Xpert MTB/RIF assay was 81%, while its specificity was 99% (8). However, a negative result does not exclude TB infection and therefore, the test should be considered a 'rule-in' rather than a 'rule-out' diagnostic tool.

In CNS tuberculomas, examination of the CSF typically reveals an elevated total protein in most patients and pleocytosis of 10–100 cells/mm^3 can be observed in approximately 50% of cases. However, it is important to note that in some instances, CSF results may remain within normal ranges.

Skin test: The diagnostic utility of the tuberculin skin test is highly variable, as it can be influenced by factors such as age, Bacillus Calmette–Guerin (BCG) vaccination, residence in high-prevalence areas, nutritional status, HIV infection, and administration technique. The test is neither sensitive nor specific for diagnosing active disease and may be helpful primarily in children.

The interferon-gamma release assay is not recommended for the diagnosis of active TB.

1.4.2 Radiological Investigations

Chest X-ray: Examine for signs of active or healed pulmonary infection.

MRI brain with contrast: In tuberculous meningitis, gadolinium-enhanced scans are more sensitive and can reveal meningeal inflammatory processes, such as meningeal enhancement over convexities, tentorium, and at basal cisterns. The common triad of findings in tuberculous meningitis includes basal meningeal enhancement (most consistent feature), hydrocephalus, and infarcts (9). In their study, Hsieh et al. identified a distinct 'TB zone' supplied by the medial striate and thalamo-perforating arteries, which was responsible for 75% of infarctions. Additionally, they found that bilaterally symmetrical infarctions within this zone were common in patients with tuberculous meningitis, occurring in 71% of cases (10).

Tuberculomas manifest with a diverse range of morphological appearances, which are contingent upon the degree of caseation. They are typically situated at the junction of the grey and white matter, and frequently exhibit a hyperintense ring on T1-weighted images, accompanied by conglomerate ring enhancement following gadolinium administration. In caseous granulomas, tuberculomas may appear hypointense on T2-weighted images, while in liquified caseation, they can exhibit hyperintensity with diffusion restriction. Moreover, tuberculomas exhibit a unique feature of 'T2 shortening', a characteristic not commonly observed in most space-occupying lesions (9). Magnetic resonance imaging can demonstrate the presence of perilesional oedema and mass effect.

CT head with contrast: CT head is helpful for diagnosing hydrocephalus, especially in an acute clinical setting. Enhancement of basal meninges can be observed on contrast studies. Tuberculomas appear hypodense or isodense on plain CT with surrounding oedema and homogenous or ring enhancement on contrast sequences.

1.5 Management

In severely ill patients, the therapeutic approach aims at patient stabilisation, management of elevated intracranial pressure, and initiation of anti-TB therapy. A systematic review and meta-analysis demonstrated that the mortality risk in tuberculous meningitis is as high as 25%, with a 51% risk of neurological sequelae (11).

1.5.1 Medical Management

Anti-TB drugs: These constitute the primary therapeutic modality for CNS infection. Treatment for suspected TB should be coordinated with the infectious disease team, and potential risk factors for drug-resistant TB should be assessed. The British Infection Society guidelines recommend first-line treatment regimen consisting of Isoniazid, RIF, Pyrazinamide, and Ethambutol for a minimum duration of 12 months for all forms of CNS TB. For RIF or Isoniazid monoresistance, quinolone can be used as a substitute and if resistant to

RIF and Isoniazid, a multi-drug-resistant TB (MDR-TB) specialist must be consulted (1).

Corticosteroids: The British Infection Society recommends the use of adjuvant corticosteroids, regardless of disease severity at presentation for tuberculous meningitis (1). The utility of corticosteroids in the management of tuberculomas remains unclear.

Anti-epileptic medications: When seizure is a presenting symptom, anti-epileptic medication should be initiated. However, there is no evidence to support the use of anti-epileptic medications prophylactically.

1.5.2 Surgical Management

Treatment of hydrocephalus: Hydrocephalus is a common sequela of tuberculous meningitis that often requires neurosurgical intervention. Nevertheless, only a subset of patients derives benefits from ventriculoperitoneal (VP) shunt surgery. To aid in diagnostic assessment, management, and prognostication, the Vellore grading system based on the Glasgow Coma Scale (GCS) (see Box 1) and management algorithm may be employed (see Figure 4) (12).

To establish tissue diagnosis: This is a more common indication for surgery with lesions suspicious for tuberculomas. In TB-endemic countries, it is common practice to initiate anti-TB therapy in patients suspected of having tuberculomas, based on clinical and radiological findings. However, in the United Kingdom, where TB prevalence is low, obtaining a tissue diagnosis is recommended to avoid unnecessary treatment and ensure proper management. Image guided biopsy may be contemplated in patients presenting with a suspected tuberculoma or abscess. In tuberculomas, histopathological examination reveals well-formed granulomas characterised by caseous necrosis, surrounded by epithelioid macrophages, Langhans giant cells, lymphocytes, and fibroblasts.

Surgical debulking of mass lesions: When the lesions are sufficiently large to generate considerable mass effect (e.g., a tuberculoma causing optic nerve compression leading to vision loss) or elevated intracranial pressure, a microsurgical debulking is a viable intervention strategy.

BOX 1 VELLORE GRADING SYSTEM OF HYDROCEPHALUS IN TUBERCULOUS MENINGITIS

Grade 1: GCS 15 with headache and no deficits
Grade 2: GCS 15 with deficits
Grade 3: GCS 9–14 with or without deficits
Grade 4: GCS-3–8 with or without deficits

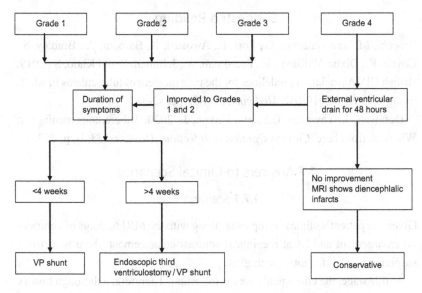

Figure 4 An algorithm for surgical decision-making in tuberculous meningitis (Adapted from (12))

1.6 Recommendations from the British Infection Society

(1) Tuberculous meningitis is a medical emergency. The empirical anti-TB therapy should be started promptly in all patients in whom the diagnosis of tuberculous meningitis is suspected as there is strong association between treatment delay and death. Do not wait for microbiological or molecular diagnostic confirmation.

(2) Diagnosis is best made by lumbar CSF. The diagnostic yield increases with the volume of CSF; repeat the lumbar puncture if the diagnosis remains uncertain.

(3) Imaging is essential for the diagnosis of cerebral tuberculoma. Attempt tissue diagnosis either by biopsy of the lesion or sampling of extra-neural sites.

(4) Treatment for all forms of CNS TB should consist of four drugs (Isoniazid, RIF, Pyrazinamide, Ethambutol) for 2 months followed by 2 drugs (Isoniazid, RIF) for at least 10 months. Adjunctive corticosteroids (either dexamethasone or prednisolone) should be given to all patients with tuberculous meningitis, regardless of disease severity.

(5) Children with CNS TB should ideally be managed by a paediatrician with familiarity and expertise in paediatric TB or otherwise with input from a paediatric infectious disease specialist.

(6) All patients with suspected or proven CNS TB should be offered testing for HIV infection.

Suggested Reading

Bracchi, M., van Halsema, C., Post, F., Awosusi, F., Barbour, A., Bradley, S., Coyne, K., Dixon-Williams, E., Freedman, A., Jelliman, P. and Khoo, S., 2019. British HIV Association guidelines for the management of tuberculosis in adults living with HIV 2019.*HIV Medicine, 20*(S6), pp. s2–s83.

Donovan, J., Thwaites, G.E. and Huynh, J., 2020. Tuberculous meningitis: Where to from here?*Current Opinion in Infectious Diseases, 33*(3), p. 259.

1.7 Answers to Clinical Scenarios

1.7.1 Scenario 1

Given the patient's clinical symptoms, along with the MRI findings of ventricular enlargement and basal meningeal contrast enhancement, there is a strong suspicion of an infectious meningitis.

At this stage, the etiological agent is uncertain. Therefore, a thorough history is essential, including recent infections, travel history, potential TB contact, the patient's occupation, and socio-economic status. Radiologically, reviewing diffusion-weighted images to look for ischemic strokes is important, as these are more common in tuberculous meningitis.

Considering the clinical presentation, the patient's neurological stability is declining. Combined with the radiological evidence suggesting a surgically addressable condition, a transfer to a neurosurgical unit for CSF diversion is imperative, as recommended by the algorithm provided in this section (see Figure 4). The local treating team was advised to arrange an urgent transfer and initiate injectable steroid therapy. (However, it is important to note that in scenarios where a patient is in critical condition and imaging reveals the presence of communicating hydrocephalus, it is advisable to promptly inform the referral team about the option of performing a lumbar puncture as a reasonable course of action. This intervention aims to reduce the elevated intracranial pressure and holds relevance in extenuating clinical situations.)

Following transfer to a tertiary-care facility, the patient underwent emergency placement of an external ventricular drain. In this case, CSF analysis provided findings consistent with tuberculous meningitis, which was confirmed via the Xpert MTB/RIF assay. Subsequently, a VP shunt was inserted, and the patient was initiated on a regimen of anti-TB therapy before being discharged.

1.7.2 Scenario 2

Given the patient's clinical history and the MRI findings suggestive of a mass lesion, we must consider a variety of differential diagnoses. The recent history of weight loss and fever, coupled with the radiological findings, raise the possibility of a metastatic brain tumour or primary brain tumour. However, considering the T2 hypointense signal in the MRI, we cannot rule out a tuberculoma.

A thorough physical examination is warranted, along with imaging studies such as a CT scan of the chest, abdomen, and pelvis. Additionally, inflammatory markers, namely CRP and ESR, should be investigated. In this case, the patient's CT scan did not reveal any abnormal findings. She underwent a craniotomy for biopsy and excision of the mass lesion. The histopathology result confirmed the diagnosis of tuberculoma.

The patient will require long-term treatment with anti-TB drugs, as advised by the local infectious disease specialist.

In rare instances, meningeal involvement may ensue secondary to the rupture of a tuberculoma into a subarachnoid space vessel. This, although exceptional, underscores the potential for complex disease progression. It's also important to consider the potential for drug resistance, in which case second-line anti-TB drugs may be needed.

Sometimes, there could be paradoxical response in intracranial tuberculomas during anti-TB therapy, likely immunological in origin, that transiently enlarges lesions and can mimic treatment non-responsiveness. This phenomenon, predominantly observed during the initial three months of treatment, can present up to two years following treatment initiation.

Lastly, the patient should be counselled about potential side effects associated with anti-TB medications to ensure they are fully informed about their treatment plan.

2 Spinal Tuberculosis Infection

2.1 Clinical Scenario

A middle-aged man presents with back pain and lower limb weakness for the past two weeks. The pain is described as a constant ache, associated with spasms and is localised to the upper back region. The patient has also noticed a gradual onset of weakness in both lower limbs, which is more pronounced on the left side, accompanied by a swelling in the back. The weakness has progressed to the point where the patient is having difficulty walking and needs support to maintain balance. The patient also reports that the pain is worse when lying on the back and is relieved by turning sideways. On physical examination, the patient has tenderness in the mid-thoracic region, and there is a loss of sensation in both lower limbs. There is also mild weakness in both lower limbs, with the left side being more affected than the right. An MRI spine with contrast was performed (see Figure 5).

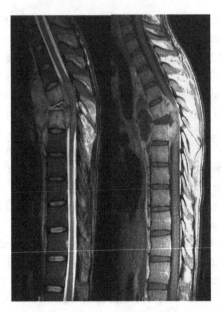

Figure 5 T2-weighted and T1-weighted with contrast MRI images

(1) What is the most likely diagnosis for a middle-aged man presenting with back pain and lower limb weakness?

(2) What additional information would you seek from the patient's medical history, physical examination, and diagnostic tests to confirm the diagnosis and assess the severity of the condition?

(3) How would you manage this patient?

(4) What factors would determine your decision for surgical intervention in this patient?

Readers can gain the necessary knowledge to manage the clinical scenario presented in this section on spinal TB and answer the questions by obtaining a comprehensive understanding of the disease.

2.2 Core Knowledge

2.2.1 Epidemiology

Spinal TB, the most common musculoskeletal TB, constitutes 50% of cases and affects 1–2% of TB patients. In 2019, the European Union/ European economic area (EU/EEA) reported 49,752 TB cases (9.6 per 100,000 population), marking a decline in the notification rate compared to 2002. Within the EU/EEA, 34.5% of TB cases were attributed to the immigrant population (13). Globally, the WHO estimated 10 million new TB cases and 1.4 million deaths in 2019.

High-burden countries, including India, Indonesia, China, Nigeria, and South Africa, accounted for 56% of new cases. The prevalence of drug-resistant TB, particularly MDR and extensively drug-resistant (XDR) TB, further complicates the epidemiology of spinal TB, emphasising the need for effective surveillance, prevention, and control measures.

2.2.2 Pathophysiology

The spread of the TB infection to the spine predominantly occurs through the haematogenous route, targeting either the paradiscal region or the vertebral body. In most of the cases (95%), the disease originates in the anterior portion of the vertebral body. The infection has a propensity to propagate subligamentously beneath the anterior longitudinal ligament and extend into the posterior vertebral body (14,15). With respect to the regional involvement of the spine, the lower thoracic spine is affected in approximately 45–50% of cases, followed by lumbar spine which accounts for 40–45%, and the cervical spine, which is involved in about 10% of cases. Various patterns of spinal involvement have been described as well (see Box 2).

2.2.3 Clinical Features

Axial back pain, associated with spine stiffness and spasms of paraspinal muscles is the most prevalent symptom which can be attributed to various causes including anterior vertebral destruction, mass effect of a cold abscess or spinal instability/deformity.

Cold abscesses represent another hallmark feature of TB infection. These abscesses typically do not elicit inflammation, often manifest in pre-/paraspinal region, becoming symptomatic due to their mass effect. In the cervical spine, a cold abscess can present as dysphagia, dyspnea, or dysphonia. In the thoracic spine, they may appear as posterior mediastinal masses, while in the lumbar spine, they can present as psoas abscess that track down to cause a swelling in the groin and thigh.

Kyphotic deformity is a late sequela resulting from anterior column destruction. Children are particularly susceptible due to their growing spine, even with complete resolution of the disease (16).

Neurological deficits can arise from either the epidural spread of abscess or spinal deformity/instability leading to canal compromise and cord compression. Cord involvement typically presents with motor and/or sensory loss in the extremities, gait imbalance, and irregularities in sphincter control.

Fever is often absent, reported in less than 40% of cases, whereas weight loss, night sweats, and malaise are manifestations that occur generally in less than 30% of patients (17).

BOX 2 PATTERNS OF SPINAL INVOLVEMENT IN SPINAL TB

- Paradiscal type: Involves the end plates around the disc and is the most common type.
- Central type: Starts in the centre of the vertebral body, spreading centrifugally leading to collapse.
- Anterior type: Involves the body along the anterior longitudinal ligament.
- Posterior type: Involves the pedicle, lamina, the articular process, or the spinous process.

2.3 Clinical Pathway

For a step-by-step guide on diagnosing and managing suspected spinal TB, the following algorithm will be helpful (see Figure 6).

2.4 Investigations

2.4.1 Laboratory Investigations

As previously discussed in this Element, laboratory investigations for suspected spinal TB are similar to those conducted for diagnosing cranial TB. For a comprehensive understanding of these investigations, please refer to Section 1.4.1.

While CSF examination is not routinely performed in spinal TB, it can be utilised in specific manifestations such as intramedullary tuberculomas or spinal tuberculous arachnoiditis.

2.4.2 Radiological Investigations

Chest X-ray: Assess for evidence of pulmonary disease.

MRI: Contrast-enhanced MRI demonstrates superior sensitivity and specificity compared to X-ray and CT. However, no pathognomonic features distinguish TB from other spinal infections or neoplasms. A whole-spine MRI is advised for detecting non-contiguous lesions, which are present in approximately 15–20% of cases.

Vertebral body involvement is typified by hypointense signals on T1-weighted images and hyperintense signals on T2-weighted sequences. Additional MRI features include relative preservation of the intervertebral disc, as well as prevertebral and paravertebral abscesses with subligamentous and epidural spread (18). Table 1 highlights some of the differences between pyogenic and tuberculous spondylodiscitis.

Tissue diagnosis: Tissue samples can be procured through CT-guided needle biopsy or surgical biopsy, particularly in urgent or expedited surgical situations.

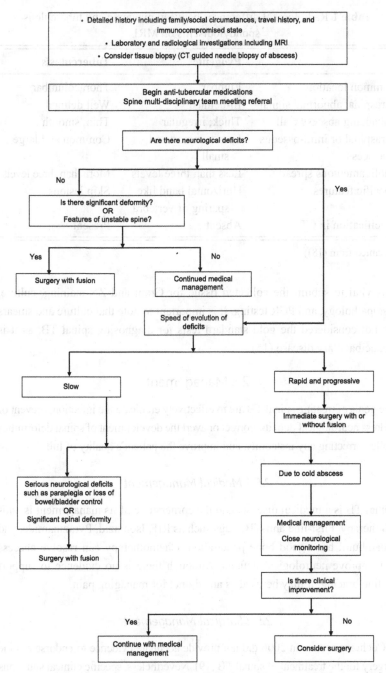

Figure 6 An algorithm for clinical approach to spinal
TB (Adapted from (15))

Table 1 Radiological differences between pyogenic and tuberculous
spondylodiscitis on MRI

	Pyogenic	**Tuberculosis**
Common location	Lumbar	Thoracolumbar
Paraspinal abnormal signal	Ill-defined	Well defined
Enhancing abscess wall	Thick, irregular	Thin, smooth
Paraspinal or intra-osseous abscess	Less common and small	Common and large
Subligamentous spread	Less than three levels	More than three levels
Specific features	Horizontal band like sparing of vertebra	Skip lesions
Calcification in CT	Absent	Present

(Adapted from (18))

It is vital to submit the collected tissue for Gram and ZN staining, culture, histopathology, and PCR testing. It is important to note that culture and smears are not considered the gold standard tests for diagnosing spinal TB, as it is a paucibacillary disease (15).

2.5 Management

The goals of treating spinal TB are to effectively eradicate the infection, prevent or address neurological deficits, correct or avert the development of spinal deformities while correcting any instability, and improve the patient's quality of life.

2.5.1 Medical Management

Spinal TB is a medical disease, and the cornerstone of its management is anti-TB therapy. First-line anti-TB drugs such as RIF, Isoniazid, Pyrazinamide, and Ethambutol have good bone penetration. Chemotherapy can resolve abscess and improve neurological deficits. Although there is no evidence to support routine bracing, it may be used as an adjunct for managing pain.

2.5.2 Surgical Management

A Cochrane review in 2006 did not provide adequate evidence to endorse routine surgery for the treatment of spinal TB (19). Nevertheless, specific clinical situations necessitate surgical intervention. Numerous surgical techniques and approaches have been described for managing spinal TB. The choice of surgical intervention can range from simple decompression to complex spinal fixations for deformity correction, which can be executed using anterior, posterior, or combined approaches. Surgical decision should be made judiciously and in the absence of clinical urgency, this decision is best made in a multidisciplinary team meeting.

Boxes 3 and 4 delineate the indications and precautions for surgical intervention in patients with TB of the spine.

Box 3 Indications for surgery in spinal TB

- Progression of neurological deficits with radiological evidence of cord compression
- Progression or persistence of disease despite adequate medical treatment
- No definite microbiological diagnosis made despite relevant investigations.
- Kyphosis more than 30 degrees
- Clinical and radiological features of instability of spine
- Cold abscess causing pressure symptoms such as dyspnea, dysphagia, or intractable pain.
- Uncertainty of diagnosis

Box 4 Precautions for surgery in TB spine

- Concomitant active pulmonary TB may be present in patients; if possible, delay surgery for two to three weeks after initiating treatment. If surgery is unavoidable, adhere to appropriate administrative, environmental controls, and utilise personal protective equipment.
- Anti-TB therapy can lead to significant side effects, such as liver enzyme induction, liver failure, peripheral neuropathy, thrombocytopenia, and blindness. Evaluate and address these factors before surgical intervention.
- Nutritional deficiencies, such as protein malnutrition or anaemia, are common in patients with TB and can negatively impact surgical outcomes. Assess and manage nutritional status preoperatively.
- Patients may exhibit restrictive pulmonary pathology or cardiac dysfunction due to severe kyphosis, which can present ventilation challenges. Airway management difficulties may arise from large prevertebral abscesses in the neck or unstable spine.
- Bony destruction in TB spine can result in spinal instability. Exercise caution during patient positioning to minimise spine displacement.
- Patients are at an elevated risk for venous thromboembolism. Implement mechanical and pharmacological prophylaxis for all patient.

Suggested Reading

Dunn, R.N. and Husien, M.B., 2018. Spinal tuberculosis: Review of current management.*The Bone & Joint Journal*, *100*(4), pp. 425–431.

Rajasekaran, S., Soundararajan, D.C.R., Shetty, A.P. and Kanna, R.M., 2018. Spinal tuberculosis: Current concepts.*Global Spine Journal*, *8*(4_suppl), pp. 96S–108S.

Tuli, S.M., 2013. Historical aspects of Pott's disease (spinal tuberculosis) management.*European Spine Journal*, *22*, pp. 529–538.

2.6 Answer to Clinical Scenario

Based on the provided clinical and radiological information, the diagnosis is likely an infectious process leading to vertebral body destruction and collapse, associated with both prevertebral and epidural abscess formation. This has resulted in significant spinal cord compression and a kyphotic deformity.

In terms of additional information, it would be pertinent to ask about fever, recent infections, immunocompromised states, socio-economic status, and history of TB exposure. The patient should undergo an infectious disease workup, including ESR, CRP, and cultures from both blood and urine. If an immunocompromised state is suspected, further investigations should be carried out as guided by infectious disease specialists. A whole spine MRI is essential to rule out any contiguous lesions, and a CT scan will provide valuable details regarding the extent of bone destruction and aids for surgical planning.

Considering the patient's progressive symptoms and spinal cord compression demonstrated on the scan, transfer to a neurosurgical centre is crucial. All spinal precautions should be meticulously followed during the transfer to prevent any exacerbation of the existing spinal cord compression or neurological worsening.

Based on the algorithm (see Figure 6), the patient would likely benefit from surgery, both for decompression and biopsy purposes. Given the severity of the deformity, an instrumented fusion would also be needed. While both anterior and posterior approaches have been described, a posterior approach was utilised in this case. The ventral epidural space can be accessed through either a transpedicular, costo-transversectomy, or lateral extracavitary route as depicted in Figure 7. Concurrently, the spinal columns can be stabilised using pedicle screws, aiming to either correct or prevent further progression of the deformity. The prevertebral abscess was not addressed surgically as it could be managed with antibiotics.

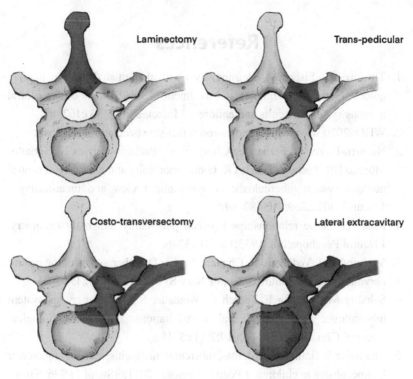

Figure 7 Posterior approaches to thoracic spine

Pus collected during the procedure was sent for culture, Gram staining, ZN staining, for Acid-Fast Bacilli, and TB PCR. Given the positive TB PCR result, the patient was initiated on anti-TB therapy.

References

1. Thwaites G, Fisher M, Hemingway C, et al. British Infection Society guidelines for the diagnosis and treatment of tuberculosis of the central nervous system in adults and children. J Infect. 2009;59(3):167–87.
2. WHO. 2020 www.who.int/news-room/fact-sheets/detail/tuberculosis.
3. Navarro-Flores A, Fernandez-Chinguel JE, Pacheco-Barrios N, Soriano-Moreno DR, Pacheco-Barrios K. Global morbidity and mortality of central nervous system tuberculosis: A systematic review and meta-analysis. J Neurol. 2022;269(7):3482–94.
4. Rich GJ. Some relationships between personality and body chemistry. J Neurol Psychopathol. 1933;14(54):132–8.
5. Muzumdar D, Vedantam R, Chandrashekhar D. Tuberculosis of the central nervous system in children. Childs Nerv Syst. 2018;34(10):1925–35.
6. Schaller MA, Wicke F, Foerch C, Weidauer S. Central nervous system tuberculosis: Etiology, clinical manifestations and neuroradiological features. Clin Neuroradiol. 2019;29(1):3–18.
7. Chatterjee S. Brain tuberculomas, tubercular meningitis, and post-tubercular hydrocephalus in children. J Pediatr Neurosci. 2011;6(Suppl 1):S96–S100.
8. Hernandez AV, de Laurentis L, Souza I, et al. Diagnostic accuracy of Xpert MTB/RIF for tuberculous meningitis: Systematic review and meta-analysis. Trop Med Int Health. 2021;26(2):122–32.
9. Bernaerts A, Vanhoenacker FM, Parizel PM, et al. Tuberculosis of the central nervous system: Overview of neuroradiological findings. Eur Radiol. 2003;13(8):1876–90.
10. Hsieh FY, Chia LG, Shen WC. Locations of cerebral infarctions in tuberculous meningitis. Neuroradiology. 1992;34(3):197–9.
11. Wang MG, Luo L, Zhang Y, et al. Treatment outcomes of tuberculous meningitis in adults: A systematic review and meta-analysis. BMC Pulm Med. 2019;19(1):1–11.
12. Rajshekhar V. Surgery for brain tuberculosis: A review. Acta Neurochir (Wien). 2015;157(10):1665–78.
13. WHO. Tuberculosis surveillance and monitoring in Europe 2021: 2019 data. 2021.
14. Garg RK, Somvanshi DS. Spinal tuberculosis: A review. J Spinal Cord Med. 2011;34(5):440–54.
15. Khanna K, Sabharwal S. Spinal tuberculosis: A comprehensive review for the modern spine surgeon. Spine J. 2019;19(11):1858–70.

16. Rajasekaran S. The natural history of post-tubercular kyphosis in children: Radiological signs which predict late increase in deformity. J Bone Joint Surg Br. 2001;83(7):954–62.

17. Trecarichi EM, Di Meco E, Mazzotta V, Fantoni M. Tuberculous spondylodiscitis: Epidemiology, clinical features, treatment, and outcome. Eur Rev Med Pharmacol Sci. 2012;16(Suppl 2):58–72.

18. Shetty A, Kanna RM, Rajasekaran S, editors. TB spine – Current aspects on clinical presentation, diagnosis, and management options. Seminars in Spine Surgery; 2016: Elsevier.

19. Jutte PC, van Loenhout-Rooyackers JH. Routine surgery in addition to chemotherapy for treating spinal tuberculosis. *Cochrane Database of Systematic Reviews.* 2006(1).

Emergency Neurosurgery

Nihal Gurusinghe
Lancashire Teaching Hospital NHS Trust

Professor Nihal Gurusinghe is a Consultant Neurosurgeon at the Lancashire Teaching Hospitals NHS Trust. He is on the Executive Council of the Society of British Neurological Surgeons as the Lead for NICE (National Institute for Health and Care Excellence) guidelines relating to neurosurgical practice. He is also an examiner for the UK and International FRCS examinations in Neurosurgery.

Peter Hutchinson
University of Cambridge, Society of British Neurological Surgeons and Royal College of Surgeons of England

Peter Hutchinson BSc MBBS FFSEM FRCS(SN) PhD FMedSci is Professor of Neurosurgery and Head of the Division of Academic Neurosurgery at the University of Cambridge, and Honorary Consultant Neurosurgeon at Addenbrooke's Hospital. He is Director of Clinical Research at the Royal College of Surgeons of England and Meetings Secretary of the Society of British Neurological Surgeons.

Ioannis Fouyas
Royal College of Surgeons of Edinburgh

Ioannis Fouyas is a Consultant Neurosurgeon in Edinburgh. His clinical interests focus on the treatment of complex cerebrovascular and skull base pathologies. His academic endeavours concentrate in the field of cerebrovascular pathophysiology. His passion is technical surgical training, fulfilled in collaboration with the Royal College of Surgeons of Edinburgh. Finally, he pursues Undergraduate Neuroscience teaching, with a particular focus on functional Neuroanatomy.

Naomi Slator
North Bristol NHS Trust

Naomi Slator FRCS (SN) is a Consultant Spinal Neurosurgeon based at North Bristol NHS Trust. She has a specialist interest in Complex Spine alongside Cranial and Spinal Trauma. She completed her neurosurgical training in Birmingham and a six-month Fellowship in CSF and Trauma (2019). She then went on to complete her Spinal Fellowship in Leeds (2020) before moving to the southwest to take up her consultant post.

Ian Kamaly-Asl
Royal Manchester Children's Hospital

Ian Kamaly-Asl is a full time paediatric neurosurgeon and Honorary Chair at Royal Manchester Children's Hospital. He trained in North Western Deanery with fellowships at Boston Children's Hospital and Sick Kids in Toronto. Ian is a member of council of The Royal College of Surgeons of England and The SBNS where he is lead for mentoring and tackling oppressive behaviours.

Peter Whitfield

University Hospitals Plymouth NHS Trust

Professor Peter Whitfield is a Consultant Neurosurgeon at the South West Neurosurgical Centre, University Hospitals Plymouth NHS Trust. His clinical interests include vascular neurosurgery, neuro oncology and trauma. He has held many roles in postgraduate neurosurgical education and is President of the Society of British Neurological Surgeons. Peter has published widely, and is passionate about education, training and the promotion of clinical research.

About the Series

Elements in Emergency Neurosurgery is intended for trainees and practitioners in Neurosurgery and Emergency Medicine as well as allied specialties all over the world. Authored by international experts, this series provides core knowledge, common clinical pathways and recommendations on the management of acute conditions of the brain and spine.

Cambridge Elements ≡

Emergency Neurosurgery

Printed in the United States
by Baker & Taylor Publisher Services

Printed in the United States
by Baker & Taylor Publisher Services